The Heart Of A Physician: Daily Devotionals for Christian Physician Assistants

Delightful Devotionals

CONTENTS

Introduction

In the fast-paced world of medicine, where each day brings new challenges and opportunities, it's essential to find moments of inspiration and connection with God. This book is crafted with the dedicated physician in mind, a healer with both scientific knowledge and a heart attuned to the greatest Physician who ever lived. As you embark on this 21-day journey, my hope is that these devotionals will serve as a guiding light, offering daily doses of encouragement, wisdom, and spiritual nourishment.

Physicians are modern-day miracle workers, equipped not only with medical expertise but also with the profound ability to bring healing and hope to those in need. This book seeks to intertwine the intricate threads of your medical journey with the timeless wisdom found in scripture. Each day, we'll explore a different aspect of your calling, from the sacred responsibility of healing hands to the resilience required in the face of challenges. Through Bible verses, reflections, and heartfelt prayers, these devotionals aim to uplift and fortify you, reinforcing the connection between your medical practice and your faith.

In the hustle and bustle of medical practice, it's easy to lose sight of the sacred nature of your work. This collection is designed to rekindle the flame of inspiration within you, reminding you of the divine purpose behind every diagnosis, treatment, and comforting word you offer.

As you open the pages of this book, may you find a source of strength, renewal, and divine connection that propels you forward in your journey as a healer and servant of humanity.

Day 1: Divine Partnerships

Verse of the Day:

Proverbs 3:6 (NIV) - "In all your ways submit to him, and he will make your paths straight."

Reflection:

As you embark on this devotional journey, consider the divine partnership you have as a physician assistant. Proverbs 3:6 reminds us to submit our ways to the Lord, trusting that He will guide our paths.

Recognize the privilege it is to work hand in hand with the Creator, using the skills and knowledge He has given you to bring healing and care to others. In your role as a physician assistant, know that you are not alone in your endeavors.

God is your ultimate partner in the journey of healing. Submit your plans and actions to Him, and find assurance in His promise to straighten your paths. Your dedication to this partnership has a profound impact on the lives you touch.

Journal:

1. Reflect on a moment in your medical career where you felt a sense of divine guidance. How did it influence your decisions and outcomes?

2. Consider the ways in which you collaborate with God in your daily work. How does acknowledging this partnership bring meaning to your role?

3. How can you enhance your reliance on God in your professional life? What steps can you take to align your ways more closely with His guidance?

Prayer:

Dear Lord, thank you for the divine partnership I have with You in my role as a physician assistant. As I submit my ways to You, grant me wisdom, discernment, and a humble heart. Guide me in my daily work, and may Your presence be evident in every interaction and decision. Amen.

Day 2: Compassion in Practice

Verse of the Day:

"Therefore, as God's chosen people, holy and dearly loved, clothe yourselves with compassion, kindness, humility, gentleness, and patience."

Reflection:

In the compassionate care you provide as a physician assistant, reflect on Colossians 3:12. Clothe yourself with compassion, for you are chosen and dearly loved by God.

Your role offers a unique opportunity to mirror God's compassion in the medical realm. As you encounter patients, colleagues, and those in need, let your actions be draped in kindness, humility, gentleness, and patience.

Embrace the understanding that your compassion is an extension of God's love. In every medical encounter, allow God's compassion to flow through you, bringing comfort and healing to those you serve.

Journal:

1. Recall a specific moment in your medical practice where you felt your compassion made a significant impact. How did it influence the outcome?

2. How can you intentionally embody compassion in your interactions with patients and colleagues? Consider practical ways to demonstrate kindness, humility, gentleness, and patience.

3. In what ways does recognizing yourself as chosen and dearly loved by God enhance your ability to show compassion? How does this perspective influence your approach to patient care?

Prayer:

Heavenly Father, I am grateful for the reminder that I am chosen and dearly loved by You. Clothe me with compassion, that I may reflect Your love in my role as a physician assistant. Grant me the strength to embody kindness, humility, gentleness, and patience in every medical encounter. May Your compassion flow through me, bringing comfort and healing to those I serve. Amen.

Day 3: Guided Wisdom

Verse of the Day:

James 1:5 (NIV) - "If any of you lacks wisdom, you should ask God, who gives generously to all without finding fault, and it will be given to you."

Reflection:

In the pursuit of accurate diagnoses and informed decisions, turn to James 1:5. Acknowledge your need for wisdom and seek it from God, who gives generously.

As a physician assistant, your role demands discernment and clarity in medical practices. Embrace the humility to recognize your dependence on God's wisdom. In challenging cases, take a moment to seek divine guidance, trusting that God provides wisdom generously.

Allow His insight to permeate your decisions, leading to improved patient care and well-informed medical practices.

Journal:

1. Recall a situation in your medical practice where seeking wisdom from God played a significant role in your decision-making. How did it impact the outcome?

2. In what ways can you incorporate intentional moments of seeking God's wisdom into your daily routine as a physician assistant?

3. How does relying on God's wisdom bring a sense of assurance and confidence in your medical decisions? Reflect on specific instances where divine guidance made a difference.

Prayer:

Dear God, I acknowledge my need for wisdom in my role as a physician assistant. Your promise in James 1:5 is a source of comfort and guidance. Grant me discernment and clarity as I navigate medical challenges. I humbly seek Your wisdom, trusting that You generously provide the insight needed for accurate diagnoses and well-informed decisions. Amen.

Day 4: Restoring Hope

Verse of the Day:

Romans 15:13 (NIV) - "May the God of hope fill you with all joy and peace as you trust in him, so that you may overflow with hope by the power of the Holy Spirit."

Reflection:

In the realm of medicine, restoring hope is a sacred mission. Romans 15:13 reminds us that our God is a God of hope, capable of filling us with joy and peace.

As a physician assistant, you play a vital role in instilling hope in patients facing medical challenges. Reflect on the privilege of being a beacon of hope, allowing the God of hope to work through you.

Trust in Him, drawing strength from the joy and peace He provides, and witness how hope overflows, bringing comfort to those in need.

Journal:

1. Think about a patient encounter where restoring hope made a significant impact. How did the presence of hope affect the patient's journey?

2. How can you, as a physician assistant, actively contribute to creating an environment of hope in your medical practice?

3. Reflect on moments when you've witnessed the power of the Holy Spirit bringing hope in challenging situations. How does this verse resonate with your experiences?

Prayer:

Heavenly Father, as I engage in the noble task of restoring hope, I pray for Your guidance. Fill me with joy and peace so that, in trusting You, I may become a vessel of hope by the power of the Holy Spirit. May Your hope overflow in the lives of those I serve. Amen.

Day 5: The Healing Touch

Verse of the Day:

Mark 5:34 (NIV) - "He said to her, 'Daughter, your faith has healed you. Go in peace and be freed from your suffering.'"

Reflection:

The healing touch holds profound significance in the realm of medicine. Mark 5:34 recounts the moment when Jesus spoke words of healing to a woman with unwavering faith.

As a physician assistant, you are an instrument of healing, contributing to the well-being of those in your care. Reflect on the impact of a compassionate touch and how faith, plays a role in the healing journey.

Embrace the privilege of being a conduit of peace and freedom from suffering through your healing touch.

Journal:

1. Recall a patient encounter where you witnessed the impact of a healing touch. How did it influence the patient's experience?

2. Consider the role of faith in the healing process. How do you navigate conversations about faith and healing with your patients?

3. Reflect on instances when you felt a sense of peace and freedom from suffering in your medical practice. How can you extend this experience to your patients?

Prayer:

Lord, grant me the wisdom and compassion to administer a healing touch that brings peace and freedom. May Your divine guidance be evident in every interaction, and may the faith of those I serve contribute to their healing. Amen.

Day 6: Balancing Act

Verse of the Day:

Proverbs 2:6 (NIV) - "For the Lord gives wisdom; from his mouth come knowledge and understanding."

Reflection:

As a physician assistant, finding the right balance between medical knowledge and faith is important. Proverbs 2:6 reminds us that wisdom comes from God. Take a moment to think about how bringing spiritual wisdom into your work makes you better at what you do.

Consider how understanding your patients not just as medical cases, but as whole people with physical, emotional, and spiritual needs, can improve your approach. Reflect on times when spiritual insights have helped you connect more deeply with patients, making your care more compassionate and complete.

Remember that the relationship between science and faith is not a conflict but a partnership. True understanding goes beyond just medical facts; it comes from a connection with the divine. This perspective can guide you to provide care that not only focuses on the body but also considers the spiritual aspect, making the healing process more meaningful.

Journal:

1. How has relying on God's wisdom influenced your decision-making in your medical practice?

2. Consider a situation where balancing medical knowledge and faith was challenging. How did you navigate it, and what did you learn?

3. Explore ways to further integrate your faith into your daily medical routines, seeking wisdom from the ultimate source.

Prayer:

Lord, grant me the wisdom to navigate the complexities of my profession. May Your understanding guide my actions, and may I find harmony in the balance between knowledge and faith. Amen.

Day 7: Strength in Challenges

Verse of the Day:

Philippians 4:13 (NIV) - "I can do all this through him who gives me strength."

Reflection:

In the face of challenges, Philippians 4:13 serves as a beacon of strength for physician assistants.

Reflect on the source of your strength and how reliance on a higher power empowers you to navigate the complexities of your medical profession.

Acknowledge that challenges are opportunities for growth and a chance to lean on the divine strength that sustains you. Embrace the confidence that, through Him, you can overcome any obstacle in your path.

Journal:

1. Identify a recent professional challenge and reflect on how your faith and inner strength helped you overcome it.

2. Consider instances where you've witnessed divine strength at work in your medical practice. How did it impact the outcome?

3. Explore ways to cultivate resilience and trust in God's strength amidst the challenges inherent in your role as a physician assistant.

Prayer:

Heavenly Father, grant me the strength to face challenges with courage and resilience. May Your power be my guide, and may I find solace in knowing that, through You, I can overcome every obstacle. Amen.

Day 8: Guided Decisions

Verse of the Day:

Isaiah 58:11 (NIV) - "The Lord will guide you always; he will satisfy your needs in a sun-scorched land and will strengthen your frame. You will be like a well-watered garden, like a spring whose waters never fail."

Reflection:

In the realm of medical decisions, guidance is paramount. As you navigate complex and often challenging situations in your role, reflect on how God's promise to guide you aligns with your experiences. Think about instances where seeking His guidance has provided clarity and direction, influencing your decisions in patient care, treatment plans, and other professional aspects.

Consider the profound impact of relying on His wisdom. In moments of uncertainty or when faced with tough choices, turning to God for guidance brings a sense of peace and strength. Ponder on specific instances where trusting in His wisdom has not only informed your decisions but also brought assurance and confidence.

Imagine your professional journey as a well-watered garden, flourishing under the guidance of God. Think about how aligning your decisions with His principles contributes to a fulfilling and fruitful practice. Recognize that, like a garden nurtured by a reliable source of water, your ability to navigate medical decisions is enhanced when rooted in the promises of His guidance.

Journal:

1. Recall a specific instance where you felt guided by God in a medical decision. How did this guidance impact the outcome?

2. In what ways can you cultivate a deeper reliance on God's guidance in your professional life?

3. Explore the concept of being a well-watered garden in your medical practice. How can you allow God's guidance to bring flourishing and satisfaction?

Prayer:

Lord, guide my decisions in my medical practice. Satisfy my needs and strengthen me, so I can be a source of healing under Your guidance. Amen.

Day 9: The Gift of Gratitude

Verse of the day:

1 Thessalonians 5:18 (NIV) - "Give thanks in all circumstances; for this is God's will for you in Christ Jesus."

Reflection:

Gratitude is a powerful and transformative gift, particularly within the demanding field of medicine. Take a moment to reflect on how cultivating gratitude aligns with God's will for you as a physician assistant. Consider the profound impact of adopting a thankful heart, not only on your personal well-being but also on your interactions with patients and colleagues.

Think about instances in your medical journey where expressing gratitude has played a role. Whether it's acknowledging a positive outcome, appreciating the collaborative efforts of a medical team, or simply being thankful for the opportunity to make a difference in someone's life, recognize how gratitude has shaped your experiences.

Consider the ripple effect of gratitude in your professional relationships.

A thankful heart often fosters a positive and compassionate environment, influencing how you connect with patients and collaborate with fellow healthcare professionals. By reflecting on the alignment of gratitude with God's will, you deepen your understanding of the transformative power of appreciation.

Journal:

1. Recall a challenging situation in your medical career. How did practicing gratitude influence your perspective on the circumstances?

2. In what ways can you incorporate intentional gratitude into your daily routine as a healthcare professional?

3. Consider the phrase "God's will for you in Christ Jesus." How does gratitude play a role in aligning your life with God's will?

Prayer:

Lord, teach me to be grateful in all circumstances. May my heart overflow with thanks, reflecting Your will in my life. Amen.

Day 10: Serving with Joy

Verse of the Day:

Psalm 100:2 (NIV) - "Worship the Lord with gladness; come before him with joyful songs."

Reflection:

In the tapestry of medicine, the threads of joy intricately weave through the fabric of service. True joy is more than a fleeting emotion; it's a disposition that can transform the healing journey for both the physician and the patient.

Consider the profound impact of approaching your medical duties with a heart brimming with joy. As you serve, let your joy be a melody that resonates with the harmonies of compassion and care.

Embrace the truth that joy is not only a reflection of a contented heart but a powerful source of strength and resilience in the demanding field of medicine.

Journal:

1. Reflect on a specific instance in your medical career when joy played a significant role in a patient's healing or in your own professional well-being.

2. How can you cultivate and sustain a joyful spirit amidst the challenges and pressures of your medical practice?

3. Explore ways in which joy can positively impact the doctor-patient relationship. How does joy contribute to a healing and supportive environment?

Prayer:

Heavenly Father, infuse my heart with the enduring joy that comes from You. May my service be a joyful song of worship, reflecting Your love and bringing comfort to those in need. Amen.

Day 11: Resilience in Medicine

Verse of the Day:

Romans 15:5 (NIV) - "May the God who gives endurance and encouragement give you the same attitude of mind toward each other that Christ Jesus had."

Reflection:

The journey of a physician is marked by the need for resilience — a steadfast spirit that withstands the storms of challenges and uncertainties. In the tapestry of medicine, resilience is not a solitary virtue but a reflection of the endurance and encouragement given by the Creator.

Consider the profound truth that your ability to endure is not solely based on personal strength but is deeply intertwined with the divine wellspring of endurance that God graciously provides.

As you navigate the complexities of medicine, lean on the enduring grace of the Almighty, drawing inspiration from the resilient spirit exemplified by Christ Jesus.

Journal:

1. Reflect on a challenging situation in your medical career where resilience played a pivotal role. How did your faith contribute to your endurance in that instance?

2. In what ways can you cultivate resilience in your daily life and medical practice? Consider both personal strategies and reliance on God's enduring strength.

3. How does the example of Christ Jesus inspire your attitude toward challenges and difficulties in your medical journey?

Prayer:

Gracious God, grant me the resilience that comes from You. In moments of difficulty, may I draw on Your enduring strength and find encouragement in Your unwavering presence. Amen.

Day 12: The Art of Listening

Verse of the Day:

James 1:19 (NIV) - "My dear brothers and sisters, take note of this: Everyone should be quick to listen, slow to speak and slow to become angry."

Reflection:

In the intricate dance of medicine, the art of listening is a melody that harmonizes with the needs and concerns of those under your care.

James encourages a posture of quick listening, deliberate speech, and measured anger—a timeless wisdom that finds resonance in the compassionate practice of medicine.

Consider the significance of truly listening, not only with ears attuned to symptoms but with a heart ready to understand the deeper narratives of those entrusted to your care. Embrace the divine art of listening, mirroring God's attentive ear to the cries of His children.

Journal:

1. Recall a moment in your medical practice where listening profoundly impacted the care you provided. How did this experience shape your understanding of the importance of listening?

2. Reflect on your current approach to listening—both to patients and colleagues. In what ways can you cultivate a deeper, more intentional practice of listening?

3. How does the biblical wisdom of being slow to speak and slow to anger resonate with the challenges you face in your medical interactions?

Prayer:

Heavenly Father, grant me the wisdom to listen with a compassionate heart. May I be quick to hear the unspoken, slow to speak words of comfort, and slow to become angry in the face of challenges. Amen.

Day 13: Embracing Diversity

Verse of the Day:

Galatians 3:28 (NIV) - "There is neither Jew nor Gentile, neither slave nor free, nor is there male and female, for you are all one in Christ Jesus."

Reflection:

In the mosaic of medicine, the concept of diversity isn't just an abstract idea; it's a vivid and beautiful reality that enriches the very fabric of healthcare. Galatians reminds us that in Christ, all distinctions fade away, and unity prevails. As a physician assistant, this biblical truth carries profound implications for your role in the medical community.

Embrace the diversity within your professional sphere, understanding that each individual's unique background and perspective contribute to the richness of the collective experience. As you navigate the varied tapestry of medical backgrounds and perspectives, consider the profound unity in diversity that reflects the essence of God's kingdom.

Just as each piece in a mosaic contributes to the overall beauty of the artwork, every individual in your medical community brings their distinctive strengths, insights, and skills. Recognize the beauty in this diversity and how it harmonizes to create a more comprehensive and compassionate approach to healthcare.

Journal

1. Consider a moment where you've witnessed the positive impact of diversity in your medical team. How did diverse perspectives contribute to better patient care?

2. Reflect on any challenges or misconceptions related to diversity that you've encountered in your medical career. How can you contribute to fostering a more inclusive environment?

3. How does the biblical truth of oneness in Christ influence your approach to patients from diverse backgrounds?

Prayer:

Gracious God, help me appreciate the beauty of diversity in my medical community. May I celebrate our unique strengths, learning from one another as we work together for the well-being of those we serve. Amen.

Day 14: Fostering Team Spirit

Verse of the Day:

Ecclesiastes 4:9 (NIV) - "Two are better than one because they have a good return for their labor."

Reflection:

In the intricate dance of medicine, collaboration is the melody that produces a harmonious outcome.

Ecclesiastes reminds us of the strength found in unity and teamwork. As a healthcare professional, cherish the bonds within your team.

Each member contributes to the collective effort, creating a more robust and effective approach to patient care.

Foster a spirit of collaboration, recognizing that together, you can achieve greater outcomes.

Journal:

1. Recall a specific instance where collaborative teamwork led to a positive patient outcome. How did each team member's contribution make a difference?

2. Consider the challenges that can arise in a healthcare team. Reflect on ways to enhance communication and teamwork in your professional setting.

3. How can you actively contribute to fostering a supportive and collaborative atmosphere within your medical team?

Prayer:

Lord, guide our healthcare team in unity and collaboration. May our combined efforts lead to the best care for our patients, reflecting the beauty of working together for a common purpose. Amen.

Day 15: A Heart for Healing

Verse of the Day:

Psalm 147:3 (NIV) - "He heals the brokenhearted and binds up their wounds."

Reflection:

In the realm of healing, it's essential to recognize that the journey extends beyond the physical aspects, encompassing the emotional and spiritual dimensions. The verse from Psalms beautifully paints a picture of God's tender care, emphasizing His capacity to heal not only physical wounds but also the deep-seated brokenness within. As a healthcare professional, especially as a physician assistant, your role is multifaceted, extending beyond the diagnosis and treatment of physical ailments.

Approach your work with a compassionate heart, acknowledging the interconnectedness of healing in its various dimensions. Just as the Divine Healer attends to the whole person, consider how you can integrate empathy and understanding into your interactions with patients. Recognize the emotional and spiritual facets of their well-being, offering not just medical expertise but a holistic approach to care.

In your daily practice, take a moment to reflect on the impact of addressing emotional and spiritual needs alongside physical concerns. Consider how your compassionate care contributes to the overall well-being of your patients, fostering an environment of healing that goes beyond the surface.

Journal:

1. Recall a moment in your medical practice where you witnessed emotional or spiritual healing in a patient. How did it impact your perspective on holistic care?

2. Consider the challenges of addressing not only physical but also emotional and spiritual needs in healthcare. How can you contribute to a more holistic approach in your field?

3. Reflect on Psalm 147:3. How does God's role as a healer of the brokenhearted inspire and guide your approach to patient care?

Prayer:

Lord, grant me the wisdom and compassion to address the holistic needs of those I serve. May my hands bring not only physical healing but also comfort to the brokenhearted. Amen.

Day 16: Nurturing Well-being

Verse of the Day:

1 Corinthians 6:19-20 (NIV) - "Do you not know that your bodies are temples of the Holy Spirit, who is in you, whom you have received from God? You are not your own; you were bought at a price. Therefore honor God with your bodies."

Reflection:

In the demanding field of medicine, where the needs of others often take precedence, it's crucial to recognize the paramount importance of your own well-being. The verse from Corinthians serves as a poignant reminder that your body is a sacred dwelling place of the Holy Spirit. Just as you dedicate yourself to nurturing the well-being of others, it's equally imperative to extend that care to yourself.

Amidst the rigors of your profession, take a moment to reflect on the divine truth encapsulated in Corinthians. Acknowledge the sanctity of your body, mind, and spirit, understanding that caring for yourself is not only a personal responsibility but also an act of honoring the divine presence within you.

As you navigate the challenges of the medical field, don't neglect your own physical, emotional, and spiritual needs. Honor God by prioritizing self-care and creating a balance that allows you to serve with excellence. Recognize that maintaining your well-being is not a luxury but a sacred duty, enabling you to fulfill your calling with vitality, compassion, and sustained dedication.

Journal:

1. Reflect on how your understanding of your body as a temple of the Holy Spirit influences your self-care practices.

2. Consider the challenges you face in maintaining a healthy work-life balance. How can you honor God with your time and energy?

3. Explore ways to integrate spiritual practices into your daily routine for personal well-being. How might this positively impact your professional life?

Prayer:

Lord, guide me in honoring you with my body and soul. Grant me the wisdom to prioritize self-care, recognizing the importance of well-being in both my personal and professional life. Amen.

Day 17: The Power of Prayer

Verse of the Day:

Philippians 4:6 (NIV) - "Do not be anxious about anything, but in every situation, by prayer and petition, with thanksgiving, present your requests to God."

Reflection:

In the midst of the intricate complexities that define the field of medicine, prayer emerges as a potent anchor. The verse from Philippians serves as an encouraging reminder to bring every concern, every patient, and every challenge before the divine presence of God.

Pause for a moment in your medical journey to reflect on the transformative power that prayer holds. Consider the peace that envelops you when you choose to entrust your cares, uncertainties, and responsibilities to the One who holds the universe in His hands.

In the fast-paced and often demanding nature of the medical profession, prayer offers a sanctuary where you can find solace, guidance, and strength beyond your own capabilities.

Embrace the profound connection that prayer fosters, recognizing that it is not just a routine but a sacred conversation with the Creator who understands the intricacies of your medical endeavors. As you navigate the challenges, may the act of prayer be a source of comfort, fortitude, and a reminder that you are not alone in your medical journey.

Journal:

1. How has prayer played a role in navigating challenging situations in your medical practice?

2. Consider specific instances where you've witnessed the impact of prayer on patient outcomes. How did it shape your perspective on the interplay between faith and medicine?

3. Explore ways to integrate prayer more intentionally into your daily routine. How might this deepen your connection with the divine in your professional life?

Prayer:

Heavenly Father, grant me the faith to surrender my concerns to You in prayer. May Your peace, which surpasses all understanding, guard my heart and mind as I continue in my medical journey. Amen.

Day 18: Humility in Service

Verse of the Day:

Verse of the Day: Philippians 2:3 (NIV) - "Do nothing out of selfish ambition or vain conceit. Rather, in humility value others above yourselves."

Reflection:

In the noble pursuit of serving others in the medical field, humility stands as a guiding principle. Take a moment to reflect on the profound wisdom encapsulated in Philippians 2:3. Consider how the practice of humility transforms your daily interactions with patients, colleagues, and the broader healthcare community.

Embrace the transformative power of humility in fostering a culture of compassion and selfless service. Humility allows you to approach each patient and situation with a teachable spirit, acknowledging the uniqueness and dignity of every individual under your care. It opens the door to collaboration, enabling you to work harmoniously with your colleagues, recognizing that each member of the healthcare team brings valuable insights and expertise.

As you navigate the intricate landscape of the medical profession, let humility be a cornerstone of your approach. It not only enhances the quality of care you provide but also contributes to a healing environment where patients feel seen, heard, and valued. In the practice of humility, you find a path to genuine connection, understanding, and a shared commitment to the well-being of those entrusted to your care.

Journal:

1. How does practicing humility influence your approach to patient care and collaboration with colleagues?

2. Consider instances where you've witnessed the impact of humility on patient outcomes. How has it shaped your understanding of effective healthcare delivery?

3. Explore practical ways to cultivate humility in your daily interactions within the medical field. How can a humble spirit enhance your effectiveness as a healthcare professional?

Prayer:

Gracious Father, instill in me the virtue of humility as I serve in the field of medicine. May my actions reflect a genuine concern for others, valuing their well-being above my own ambitions. Guide me in humility as I strive to make a positive impact on those entrusted to my care. Amen.

Day 19: Facing Uncertainties

Verse of the Day:

Proverbs 16:9 (NIV) - "In their hearts humans plan their course, but the Lord establishes their steps."

Reflection:

In the unpredictable journey of medicine, uncertainties abound, and it's in these moments of ambiguity that Proverbs 16:9 provides a comforting anchor. Take a moment to reflect on the profound wisdom of this verse and find solace in the divine assurance that, even in the face of uncertainty, God is orchestrating our steps.

Embrace the humility to acknowledge the limits of human planning. In the intricate tapestry of medical decisions and unforeseen challenges, entrust your path to the One who holds the future. This acknowledgment of God's sovereign guidance invites a sense of peace, allowing you to navigate uncertainties with a spirit of trust and assurance.

As you encounter the unpredictability inherent in the medical profession, let the wisdom of Proverbs 16:9 be a source of encouragement. Embrace the divine order that surpasses human understanding, finding strength in the assurance that your journey is guided by a loving and purposeful hand.

Journal:

1. How do you navigate uncertainties in your medical practice? Reflect on past experiences where God's guidance became evident in unexpected situations.

2. Consider the balance between strategic planning and surrendering to God's guidance. In what ways can you align your aspirations with His overarching plan?

3. Explore the concept of faith in the context of facing uncertainties. How can cultivating trust in God impact your mindset and actions in the medical field?

Prayer:

Heavenly Father, in the face of uncertainties, I turn to You for guidance. Establish my steps as I navigate the complexities of medicine. Grant me the wisdom to discern Your leading and the faith to trust in Your divine plan. Amen.

Day 20: Inspiring Innovation

Verse of the Day:

Exodus 31:3 (NIV) - "I have filled him with the Spirit of God, with wisdom, with understanding, with knowledge and with all kinds of skills."

Reflection:

God's divine infusion of wisdom, understanding, knowledge, and skills empowers innovation. Take a moment to reflect on the profound truth embedded in Exodus 31:3, acknowledging that your abilities are gifts from the Creator Himself.

Embrace the challenge to inspire innovation in your medical practice, recognizing that your unique set of skills and insights is part of a divine plan. Trust in the Spirit's guidance as you navigate the complexities of healthcare, allowing your innovative spirit to be a reflection of the creativity instilled in you by the Divine.

As you explore new ways to enhance patient care, improve processes, or contribute to medical advancements, let the wisdom of Exodus 31:3 be a driving force. Recognize that your innovative pursuits are not only a manifestation of your God-given talents but also an opportunity to participate in the ongoing work of creation. Trust in the Spirit's guidance, knowing that your commitment to innovation is aligned with the Creator's plan for healing and restoration.

Journal:

1. Consider instances where innovation played a role in medical advancements. How can you foster a spirit of innovation in your work?

2. Reflect on the diverse skills and knowledge you possess. In what ways can you leverage these gifts to bring positive change in your medical community?

3. Explore the intersection of faith and creativity. How might your spiritual perspective contribute to innovative approaches in medicine?

Prayer:

Gracious God, fill me with Your Spirit, igniting creativity and innovation in my medical endeavors. Grant me the wisdom to use my skills for the betterment of others and the glory of Your name. Amen.

Day 21: Divine Dedication

Verse of the Day:

Colossians 3:23-24 (NIV) - "Whatever you do, work at it with all your heart, as working for the Lord, not for human masters, since you know that you will receive an inheritance from the Lord as a reward. It is the Lord Christ you are serving."

Reflection:

In the dedication of your work, remember that you serve the Lord. Take a moment to reflect on the profound truth encapsulated in Colossians 3:23-24, recognizing your labor as a sacred offering to God Himself.

As a medical professional, your commitment to excellence and compassionate care is not merely a job but a sacred calling. Consider how your daily efforts in serving others align with the divine call to work with all your heart. Whether you're attending to patients' needs, conducting research, or contributing to the overall well-being of your community, see each task as an opportunity to glorify God through your dedication.

Embrace the understanding that your work, done with diligence and love, is a form of worship. In every interaction, let the principles of Colossians 3:23-24 guide you, infusing your medical practice with a sense of purpose and devotion. Your service is not just to individuals in need but, ultimately, to the Lord Christ, whose love and grace flow through you to bring healing and hope to those you serve.

Journal:

1. How does the idea of working for the Lord impact your approach to daily tasks in your medical profession?

2. Reflect on moments when your dedication to your work has made a positive impact on others. How did it align with your commitment to serve Christ?

3. Consider the challenges you face in your medical career. How can a mindset of divine dedication bring purpose and fulfillment to your work?

Prayer:

Heavenly Father, may my work be a dedication to You, done with all my heart. Guide me in serving others with compassion and excellence, knowing that, ultimately, I serve You. Amen.

Conclusion

As we conclude this transformative journey through this book, I want to express my heartfelt gratitude for sharing these moments of reflection and inspiration. Over these 21 days, we've explored the intricate balance of science and faith, the challenges you face as a healer, and the profound impact of your dedication on the lives you touch.

In the realm of medicine, where the demands are high and the stakes even higher, it's crucial to pause, reflect, and connect with the divine source of strength. This book aimed to be a companion on your journey, providing a daily oasis of encouragement and a reminder of the sacredness embedded in your role as a physician assistant.

Remember, your healing hands are not merely instruments of science but vessels of grace. As you continue to navigate the complexities of the medical field, may you carry with you the wisdom gleaned from these devotionals.

May the resilience, compassion, and dedication that have been highlighted in these pages serve as a continuous wellspring of inspiration in your practice.

It is my sincerest hope that this devotional journal has been a source of empowerment, encouragement, and a testament to the divine calling embedded in your profession. May you continue to find strength in your faith, joy in your service, and fulfillment in the remarkable impact you make. May your journey be filled with God's guidance, and may your healing hands be a conduit of His love in every patient encounter.

With warmest wishes and gratitude,

Delightful Devotionals